Emergency
First Aid
Made Easy

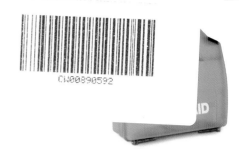

Introduction

This booklet has been designed by an experienced paramedic instructor to guide you through your first aid course and to provide you with a quick reference for future years.

Effective emergency treatment before professional help arrives can go a long way to reducing the effects of illness and injury and indeed save someone's life.

Taking part in a first aid course and using this book may be the most important decision you make in your life…

Edition 6.1

Important

This book is designed as a learning guide to a full first aid course and cannot replace hands-on training in the skills of dealing with an emergency situation.

The circumstances in which illness and injury occur vary considerably and are outside the control of the author, so it is not possible to give definitive guidance for every situation. If you suspect illness or injury therefore, you should always seek immediate professional medical advice.

Whilst every effort has been made to ensure the accuracy of the information contained within this book, the author does not accept any liability for any inaccuracies or for any subsequent mistreatment of any person, however caused.

Contents

Priorities of treatment – Primary survey

All animal life needs a constant supply of oxygen to survive. If the oxygen doesn't get through, brain cells will start to die within 3 to 4 minutes. The priorities of treatment are therefore aimed at ensuring oxygen gets into the blood, ensuring that the blood is circulating around the body, and preventing the loss of that blood.

The Primary Survey is a fast and systematic way to find and treat any life-threatening conditions in a priority order. As a life-threatening condition is found, it should be treated immediately, then you should move on to the next step in the survey.

Perform a primary survey first on every casualty you treat and until it's complete, do not be distracted by more superficial, non-life-threatening conditions.

Multiple casualties

Use the DRABC primary survey to decide who needs treatment first. A rough rule of thumb is that the casualty who is the quietest needs treatment first, whereas the one making the most noise (trying to get your attention) is the least serious!

Use DRABC ('*Doctor ABC*') to remember the primary survey sequence.

 Danger

- Ensure that the casualty, any bystanders and you are safe.

 Response

- Quickly check to see if the casualty is conscious. Gently shake or tap the shoulders and ask loudly 'are you alright?'
- Unconscious casualties take priority and need urgent treatment.

 Airway

- Identify and treat any life-threatening airway problems (*such as choking or suffocation*).
- If the casualty is unconscious, tilt the head to open the airway.
- When the airway is clear/opened, move on to **Breathing**:

 Breathing

- Identify and treat any life-threatening breathing problems (*such as asthma*).
- If the casualty is unconscious and not breathing normally, perform CPR (*see pages 4–6*). Once you start CPR, you are unlikely to move on to the next step in the primary survey.
- When life-threatening breathing problems have been ruled out or treated, move on to **Circulation**.

 Circulation

- Identify and treat any life-threatening circulation problems (*such as severe bleeding or heart attack*).
- When life-threatening circulation problems have been ruled out or treated, the primary survey is complete. You can now perform a **Secondary Survey** (*page 9*) to look for other conditions (*such as broken bones*).

The following flow chart puts the DRABC Primary Survey into action in the context of a casualty who needs resuscitation *(note that at 'Breathing' CPR is started, so 'Circulation' is not reached).*

Remove Danger

Make the scene safe.

Do not take risks.

YES

DANGER?
Look for any further danger.

NO

RESPONSE?
Shout and gently shake or tap the casualty.

NO

Help!
Shout for help but don't leave the casualty yet.

AIRWAY
Open the airway by tilting the head back and lifting the chin.

Normal BREATHING?
Look, listen and feel for no more than 10 seconds.

If you're not sure if breathing is normal, treat it as though it is **not.**

NO

Call 999/112 Now
(If not already done).

Resuscitation

30 to 2

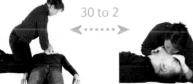

- Give 30 chest compressions, then 2 rescue breaths.
- Continue giving cycles of 30 compressions to 2 rescue breaths.
- Only stop to recheck the casualty if they start to regain consciousness AND start breathing normally.
- If there is more than one rescuer, change over every 1–2 minutes to prevent fatigue.

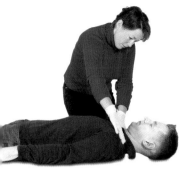

Gently shake the shoulders and shout.

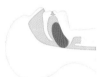

Airway blocked by the tongue

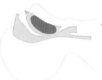

Airway cleared by tilting the head

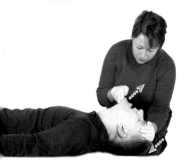

Tilt the head back and lift the chin to open the airway.

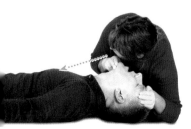

Look, listen and feel for normal breathing.

Resuscitation

 D **Danger**

- Make sure that the casualty, any bystanders and you are safe.

 R **Response**

- Gently shake the shoulders and ask loudly 'Are you alright?'
- If they respond, keep them still, find out what's wrong and get help if needed.
- If there is no response, shout for help immediately, but do not leave the casualty yet.

 A **Airway**

- Carefully open the airway by using 'head tilt' and 'chin lift':
  - Place your hand on the forehead and gently tilt the head back.
  - With your fingertips under the point of the casualty's chin, lift the chin to open the airway *(see picture)*.

B **Breathing**

Keeping the airway open, check to see if the breathing is normal. Take no more than 10 seconds to do this:

- **Look** for chest movement.
- **Listen** at the mouth for breathing sounds.
- **Feel** for air on your cheek.

WARNING: In the first few minutes after cardiac arrest, a casualty may be barely breathing, or taking infrequent, noisy gasps. These are known as 'agonal' gasps – do not confuse this with normal breathing.
If you are in doubt, start CPR.

If the casualty **is** breathing **normally**, place them in the recovery position *(page 10)*, then complete the primary and secondary surveys *(pages 2 and 9)*.

Continued on next page.

If the casualty is not breathing normally:

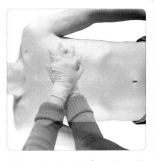

Ask someone to **call for an ambulance and bring a defibrillator (AED)** if available.

If you are on your own, use your mobile phone to call if possible. Only leave the casualty if there is no other way of obtaining help.

Kneel at the side of the casualty and start chest compressions as follows:

- Place the heel of one hand in the centre of the casualty's chest, then place the heel of your other hand on top and interlock your fingers *(see picture)*.

Place the heel of one hand in the centre of the chest, then the other hand on top.

- Position yourself vertically above the casualty's chest with your arms straight.
- Press down on the breastbone 5–6cm, then release all the pressure without losing contact between your hands and the chest *(chest compression)*. Avoid applying pressure over the casualty's ribs, the bottom end of the breastbone or the upper abdomen.
- Compression and release should take an equal amount of time.
- **Do 30 chest compressions** at a rate of 100–120 per minute.
- Now combine chest compressions with rescue breaths *(overleaf)*.

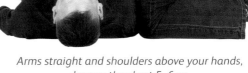

Arms straight and shoulders above your hands, depress the chest 5–6cm.

Now combine chest compressions with rescue breaths – *over the page*

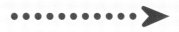

NOTE: Ideally the casualty needs to be on a firm flat surface to perform chest compressions (not a bed). One way to remove someone from a low bed is to unhook the bed sheets and use them to slide the casualty carefully to the floor. Get help if you can and be very careful not to injure yourself or the casualty. If you think it's too risky to move the casualty, attempting CPR on the bed is better than no CPR at all (remove the pillows).

Combine chest compressions with rescue breaths:

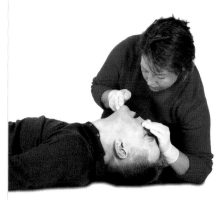

Nip the nose.

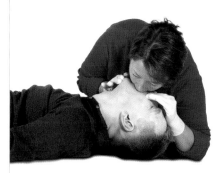

Rescue breaths.

- Open the airway again, then nip the soft part of the casualty's nose closed. Allow the mouth to open, but maintain chin lift.

- Take a normal breath and seal your lips around the casualty's mouth.

- Blow steadily into the casualty's mouth, whilst watching for the chest to rise *(rescue breath)*. Take about one second to make the chest rise.

- Keeping the airway open, remove your mouth. Take a normal breath of fresh air and watch for the casualty's chest to fall as air comes out.

- Re-seal your mouth and give another rescue breath *(two in total)*. Giving both rescue breaths should not take more than 5 seconds.

- Return your hands without delay to the centre of the chest and give another 30 chest compressions *(then 2 more rescue breaths)*.

- **Continue repeating cycles of 30 chest compressions and 2 rescue breaths.**

- Only stop to recheck the casualty if they show signs of regaining consciousness *(see below)* AND start to breathe normally – otherwise **do not interrupt resuscitation**.

*NOTE: If there is more than one rescuer present, another should take over CPR every one to two minutes to prevent fatigue. Ensure the minimum of delay during changeover and **do not interrupt chest compressions**.*

If the initial rescue breath in each sequence does not make the chest rise *(as in normal breathing)*, give another 30 chest compressions, then before your next attempt:

- Check the casualty's mouth and remove any visible obstruction.
- Recheck that there is adequate head tilt and chin lift.
- Do not attempt more than two breaths each time before returning to chest compressions.

Continue resuscitation until:

- Qualified help arrives and takes over.
- You become exhausted, OR
- The casualty shows signs of regaining consciousness *(such as coughing, opening eyes, speaking or moving purposefully)* AND starts to breathe normally.

Resuscitation for children and babies

Recent studies have found that many children do not receive resuscitation because potential rescuers fear causing them harm. It is important to understand that it's far better to perform 'adult style' resuscitation on a child (who is unresponsive and not breathing) than to do nothing at all.

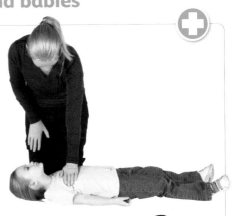

For ease of learning and retention, first aiders can use the adult sequence of resuscitation (see previous pages) on a child or baby who is unresponsive and not breathing. The following minor modifications to the adult sequence will, however, make it even more suitable for use in children:

- Give **five** initial rescue breaths before starting chest compressions (then continue at the ratio of **30** compressions to **2** breaths).

- If you are on your own, perform resuscitation for about 1 minute before going for help.

- Compress the chest by at least one-third of its depth:

  - For a baby under 1 year, use **two fingers.**

  - For a child over 1 year, use **one or two hands** as required to depress the chest at least a third of its depth.

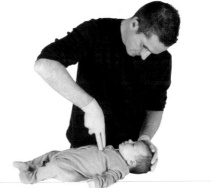

Chest compression only resuscitation

When an adult casualty suffers a cardiac arrest, it is likely that there is residual oxygen left in the blood stream.

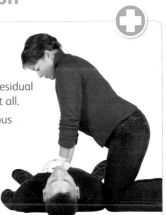

If you are not trained (or unwilling) to give rescue breaths, give 'chest compressions only' resuscitation, as this will circulate any residual oxygen in the blood stream, so it is better than no resuscitation at all.

- If chest compressions only are given, these should be continuous at a rate of 100–120 per minute.

- Stop to recheck the casualty only if they start to regain consciousness AND start breathing normally – otherwise do not interrupt resuscitation.

- If there is more than one rescuer, change over every one to two minutes to prevent fatigue. Ensure the minimum of delay as you change over.

Vomiting

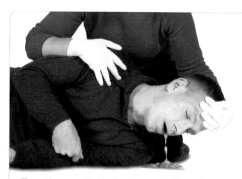

It is common for a casualty who has stopped breathing to vomit whilst they are collapsed. This is a passive action in the unconscious person, so you may not hear or see it happening. You might not find out until you give a rescue breath *(as the air comes back out of the casualty it makes gurgling noises)*.

- If the casualty has vomited, turn them onto their side, tip the head back and allow the vomit to run out.
- Clean the face of the casualty then continue resuscitation, using a protective face barrier if possible.

Turn them onto their side and allow the vomit to run out.

Hygiene during resuscitation

- Wipe the lips clean.
- If possible use a protective barrier such as a 'face shield' or 'pocket mask'. *(This is particularly important if the casualty suffers from any serious infectious disease such as TB, Hepatitis or S.A.R.S.).*
- As a last resort some plastic with a hole in it, or a handkerchief, may help to prevent direct contact.
- If you are still in doubt about the safety of performing rescue breaths, give 'chest compression only' resuscitation *(see page 7)*.
- Wear protective gloves if available and wash your hands afterwards.

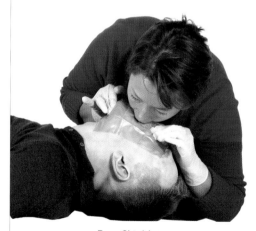

Face Shield

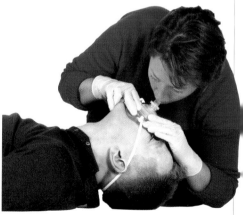

Pocket Mask

Using a protective barrier during CPR.

Secondary Survey

When the primary survey is complete *(page 2)* and you have dealt with any life-threatening conditions, it is safe to examine the casualty head to toe, checking for other injuries or illnesses in a methodical manner. This assessment can be carried out on a conscious or unconscious casualty. Start by considering the:

History   What happened? Is the casualty likely to have injuries?

Signs   Clues such as swelling, pale skin, deformity etc.

Symptoms   How does the casualty feel? Do they have any pain?

Head to toe examination

Next check the casualty from head to toe. Protect dignity and ask permission if possible. Wear disposable gloves and do not move the casualty more than necessary.

Protecting the airway takes priority *(page 2)*, so if a casualty is unconscious and breathing, but you are concerned about the airway for any reason *(e.g. vomiting)* place them in the recovery position immediately *(page 10)*. If a casualty is already in the recovery position, perform the check with them in that position.

Head and neck   Assess the breathing and the pulse – is it normal? Check the size of the pupils *(page 23)*. Check the whole head and face. Clues to injury could be bruising, swelling, deformity, bleeding or discharge from the ear or nose. Has the casualty had an accident that might have injured the neck? *(page 21)*.

Shoulders and chest   Compare opposite shoulders and collar bones. Are there signs of a fracture? *(page 20)*. Ask a conscious casualty to take a deep breath. Does the chest move easily and equally on both sides? Does this cause pain? Feel the rib cage at either side and compare. Look for injuries such as stab wounds or bleeding.

Abdomen and pelvis   Gently feel the abdomen. Check for abnormality or response to pain. Look for incontinence or bleeding.

DO NOT squeeze or rock the pelvis.

Legs and arms   Check each leg and then each arm for the signs of a fracture or deformity. Ask a conscious casualty if they can move their arms, legs and all the joints without causing pain.

Pockets and clues   Check for clues and have a reliable witness if you remove items from pockets. Be very careful if you suspect there could be sharp objects such as needles. Look for other clues *(medic alert bracelets, needle marks, medication etc)*. Loosen any tight clothing.

The recovery position

When a person is unconscious and lying on their back, the airway can become compromised by the **tongue** touching the back of the throat, or **vomit** if the casualty is sick. Placing the casualty in the recovery position protects the airway from both of these dangers – the tongue will not fall backwards and vomit will run out of the mouth.

1

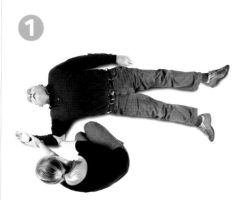

2

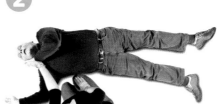

- Remove the casualty's glasses and straighten both legs.
- Move the arm nearest you outwards, elbow bent with palm uppermost.

- Bring the far arm across the chest, and hold the back of that hand against the cheek.

3

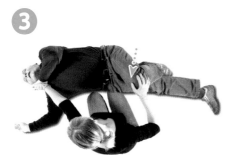

4

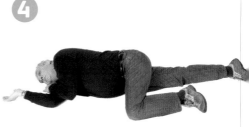

- With your other hand, grasp the far leg just above the knee, and pull it up, keeping the foot on the ground.
- Keeping the casualty's hand pressed against their cheek, pull on the leg to roll them towards you, onto their side.

- Adjust the upper leg so that the hip and knee are bent at right angles and tilt the head back to keep the airway open.
- **Call 999/112 for emergency help.**
- Check breathing regularly. If you are in any doubt about the presence of normal breathing, start CPR (see page 4).

Choking – ADULT

Firstly, encourage the casualty to cough. If the choking is only mild, this will clear the obstruction and the casualty should be able to speak to you.

If the obstruction is not cleared:

1 Back blows

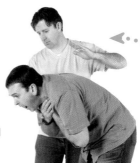

- **Shout for help**, but don't leave the casualty yet.
- Bend the casualty forwards so the head is lower than the chest.
- Give up to 5 firm blows between the shoulder blades with the palm of your hand. Check between blows and stop if you clear the obstruction.

If the obstruction is still not cleared:

2 Abdominal thrusts

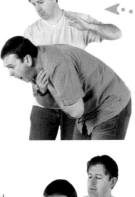

- Stand behind the casualty. Place both your arms around their waist.
- Make a fist with one hand and place it just above the belly button *(below the ribs)* with your thumb inwards.
- Grasp this fist with your other hand, then pull sharply inwards and upwards. Do this up to 5 times. Check between thrusts and stop if you clear the obstruction.

If the obstruction is still not cleared:

3 Repeat steps 1 and 2

- Keep repeating steps 1 and 2.
- If the treatment seems ineffective, shout for help. Ask someone to **call 999/112 for emergency help**, but don't interrupt the treatment whilst the casualty is still conscious.

If the casualty becomes unconscious

- Support the casualty carefully to the ground and immediately **call 999/112 for emergency help** *(if not already done)*.
- **Start CPR** – follow the sequence on page 5 after the heading 'if the casualty is not breathing normally:'

After successful treatment, any casualty who has received abdominal thrusts, with a persistent cough, difficulty swallowing or with the feeling of an 'object still stuck in the throat' should seek immediate medical attention.

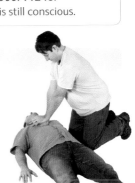

If the casualty becomes unconscious – start CPR.

Choking – CHILD *(over 1 year)*

Firstly encourage the child to cough. If the choking is only mild, this will clear the obstruction and the child should be able to speak to you.

If the obstruction is not cleared:

1 Back blows

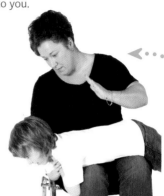

- **Shout for help,** but don't leave the child yet.
- Lean the child over your knee or bend them forwards, so the head is lower than the chest.
- Give up to 5 firm blows between the shoulder blades with the palm of your hand. Check between blows and stop if you clear the obstruction.

If the obstruction is still not cleared:

2 Abdominal thrusts

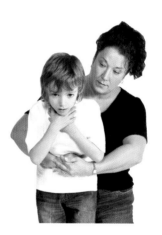

- Kneel or stand behind the child. Place both your arms around their waist.
- Make a fist with one hand, and place it just above the belly button *(below the ribs)* with your thumb inwards. Grasp this fist with your other hand.
- Thrust sharply inwards and upwards. Try this up to 5 times. Check between thrusts and stop if you clear the obstruction.

If the obstruction is still not cleared:

3 Repeat steps 1 and 2

- Keep repeating steps 1 and 2.
- If the treatment seems ineffective, shout for help. Ask someone to **call 999/112 for emergency help,** but don't interrupt the treatment whilst the child is still conscious.

If the child becomes unconscious

- Place the child on a firm, flat surface.
- **START CPR** – *(pages 4–7).*

NOTE: information on when to seek medical attention is on page 11.

Choking – BABY *(under 1 year)*

The baby may attempt to cough. If the choking is only mild, this will clear the obstruction – the baby may cry and should now be able to breathe effectively.

If the obstruction is not cleared:

1 Back blows

- **Shout for help**, but don't leave the baby yet.
- Lay the baby over your arm, face down, legs either side of your elbow with the head below the chest *(see picture)*.
- Give up to 5 blows between the shoulder blades with the palms of your fingers. Keeping the head low, check between blows and stop if you clear the obstruction.

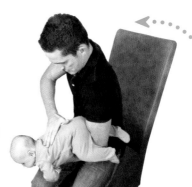

If the obstruction is still not cleared:

2 Chest thrusts

- Turn the baby over, chest uppermost, *(by laying them on your other arm)* and lower the head below the level of the chest.
- Using two fingers on the chest, give up to 5 chest thrusts. These are similar to chest compressions, but sharper in nature and delivered at a slower rate. Keeping the head low, check between thrusts and stop if you clear the obstruction.

NEVER perform abdominal thrusts on a baby.

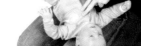

If the obstruction is still not cleared:

3 Repeat steps 1 and 2

- Keep repeating steps 1 and 2.
- If the treatment seems ineffective, shout for help. Ask someone to **call 999/112 for emergency help**, but don't interrupt the treatment whilst the baby is still conscious.

If the baby becomes unconscious

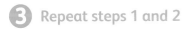

- Place the baby on a firm, flat surface.
- **START CPR** – *(pages 4–7)*.

NOTE: information on when to seek medical attention is on page 11.

How much blood do we have?

The amount of blood in our body varies in relation to our size, so a child or baby will have much less blood than an adult.

A rough rule of thumb is that a person has approximately one pint of blood per stone in body weight *(0.5 litres per 7kg)* but the rule doesn't work for someone who is overweight.

How much blood loss is critical?

The body can compensate if it is losing blood. It does this by:

- Closing down the blood supply to non-emergency areas of the body *(including the skin and digestive system).*
- Speeding up the heart to maintain blood pressure.

Blood vessels can only close down so much, and the heart can only go so fast, so there is a limit to the amount of blood loss the body can compensate for. The body can no longer compensate after **one third** of its blood has been lost. After this amount, the blood pressure will fall quickly, the blood supply to the brain will fail and death will result.

Particular care is needed for a child who has lost blood, because one third of their blood supply will be much less than that of an adult. The critical blood loss for a baby weighing one stone for example, is just one third of a pint!

Shock

The definition of shock is *'a lack of oxygen to the tissues of the body, usually caused by a fall in blood volume or blood pressure'.*

Severe bleeding can result in shock, which can kill. If the casualty has lost a large quantity of blood this can cause a reduction in blood supply to the brain *(don't forget that children can't afford to lose as much blood as adults!).*

Some signs of shock are:

- Pale clammy skin *(with blue or grey tinges if it's severe).*
- Dizziness or passing out *(especially if they try to stand or sit up).*
- A fast, weak pulse.
- Rapid shallow breathing.

If a large amount of blood has been lost, you can help the flow of blood to the brain by laying the casualty down and raising their legs. Keep the casualty warm *(but don't overheat them)*, give nothing by mouth and **call 999/112 for emergency help.**

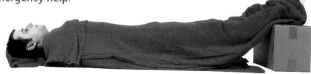

Internal bleeding

Internal bleeding is a serious condition, yet it can be very difficult to recognise in its early stages. Severe internal bleeding can result from injuries to the upper leg, pelvis, abdomen or a lung.

Suspect internal bleeding after an accident if the signs of shock develop *(opposite)*, yet there is no other obvious cause *(such as external bleeding)*.

- **Call 999/112 for emergency help and treat the casualty for shock as necessary.**

Treatment of bleeding

The aims of treatment for external bleeding are firstly to stop the bleeding, to prevent the casualty from going into shock *(opposite)* and then to prevent infection.

S.E.E.P. will help you to remember the steps of treatment:

S Sit or lay Sit or lay the casualty down. Place them in a position that is appropriate to the location of the wound and the extent of their bleeding.

E Examine Examine the wound. Look for foreign objects and note how the wound is bleeding. Remember what it looks like, so you can describe it to medical staff when it's covered with a bandage.

E Elevate Elevate the wound. Ensure that the wound is above the level of the heart, using gravity to reduce the blood flow to the injury.

P Pressure Apply direct pressure over the wound to stem the bleeding. If there is an embedded object in the wound, you may be able to apply pressure at either side of the object.

ALWAYS wear protective gloves when dealing with wounds and bleeding!

Dressings

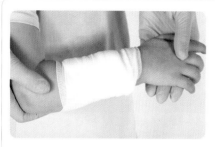

A dressing should be sterile and just large enough to cover the wound. It should be absorbent and preferably made of material that won't stick to the clotting blood (a 'low-adherent' dressing).

A firmly applied dressing is sufficient to stem bleeding from the majority of minor wounds, but the dressing should not restrict blood flow to the rest of the limb (check the circulation at the far side of the dressing).

Extra pressure 'by hand' and elevation may be necessary for severe bleeding. If the dressing becomes saturated with blood, keep it in place and put another larger dressing on top. If this doesn't work take the dressings off and start again. Make sure you apply pressure and elevate the wound.

For a hand or arm wound it is a good idea to place the arm in an elevated sling after you have dressed it.

NEVER try to stop bleeding by tying a band around the limb (a tourniquet). It may cause tissue damage or make the bleeding worse.

NEVER remove an embedded object (other than a splinter). It may be stemming bleeding and further damage may result.

Eye injury

Small particles of dust or dirt can be washed out of an eye with cold tap water. Ensure the water runs away from the good eye.

For a more serious eye injury:

- Keep the casualty still and gently hold a soft sterile dressing over the injured eye. This can be carefully bandaged in place if necessary.
- Tell the casualty to close their good eye, because any movement of this will cause the injured eye to move also. If necessary bandage the good eye to stop the casualty using it. Lots of reassurance will be needed!
- Take the casualty to hospital. **Call 999/112 for emergency help** if necessary.

For chemicals in the eye:

- Wear protective gloves. Wash with copious amounts of clean water, ensuring the water runs away from the good eye. Gently but firmly try to open the casualty's eyelid to irrigate the eye fully. **Call 999/112 for emergency help**.

Amputation

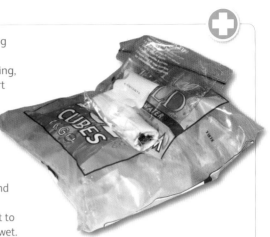

Amputation is the complete or partial severing of a limb, and is extremely traumatic for the casualty. Your priorities are to stop any bleeding, to carefully preserve the amputated body part and to reassure the casualty.

- Treat the casualty for bleeding *(page 15)*.
- **Call 999/112 for emergency help.**
- Dress the wound with a 'low-adherent', non-fluffy dressing.
- Place the amputated part in a plastic bag and then put the package on a bag of ice to preserve it. Do not allow the amputated part to come into direct contact with the ice or get wet.

Embedded objects

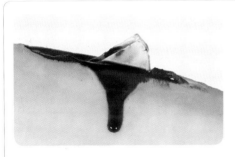

Objects embedded in a wound:

An object embedded in a wound *(other than a small splinter)* should not be removed as it may be stemming bleeding, or further damage may result.

Use sterile dressings and bandages to 'build up' around the object. This will apply pressure around the wound and support the object. Send the casualty to hospital to have the object removed.

Splinters:

If a splinter is embedded deeply, difficult to remove or on a joint, leave it in place and follow the advice for embedded objects above. Other splinters can be removed as follows:

- Carefully clean the area with warm soapy water.
- Using a pair of clean tweezers, grip the splinter as close to the skin as possible. Gently pull the splinter out at the same angle that it entered.
- Gently squeeze around the wound to encourage a little bleeding. Wash the wound again, then dry and cover with a dressing.
- Seek medical advice to ensure the casualty's tetanus immunisation is up-to-date.

Objects embedded in the nose, ear or other orifice:

Do not attempt to remove anything that someone has got stuck in their ear, nose or other orifice. Take them to hospital where the professionals can remove it safely.

Nosebleed

Weakened or dried out blood vessels in the nose can rupture as a result of a bang to the nose, picking or blowing it. More serious causes of a nosebleed could be high blood pressure or a fractured skull.

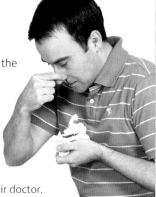

- Sit the casualty down, head tipped forward.
- Nip the soft part of the nose. Maintain constant pressure for 10 minutes.
- Tell the casualty to breathe through the mouth.
- Give the casualty a disposable cloth to mop up any blood whilst the nose is nipped.
- Advise the casualty not to breathe through the nose for a few hours. Avoid blowing or picking the nose and hot drinks for 24 hours.
- If bleeding persists for more than 30 minutes, or if the casualty takes 'anti-coagulant' drugs *(such as warfarin)*, take or send them to hospital in an upright position.
- Advise a casualty suffering from frequent nosebleeds to visit their doctor.

Poisoning

A poison can either be:

Corrosive   Such as: acids, bleach, ammonia, petrol, turpentine, dishwasher powder, etc.

OR

Non-Corrosive   Such as: tablets, drugs, alcohol, plants, perfume etc.

NEVER make the casualty vomit. This may put the airway in danger.

For a corrosive substance:

- Don't endanger yourself – make sure it's safe to help.
- Dilute the substance or wash it away if possible:
  - Substances on the skin – wash away with water *(see burns)*.
  - Swallowed substances – get the casualty to rinse out their mouth, then give frequent sips of milk or water.
- **Call 999/112 for emergency help**. Give information about the poison if possible. Take advice from the ambulance operator.

For a non-corrosive substance:

- **Call 999/112 for emergency help**. Give information about the poison if possible. Take advice from the ambulance operator.

It helps the Paramedics if you:

- *Pass on containers, or other information about the substance.*
- *Find out how much has been taken.*
- *Find out when it was taken.*
- *Keep samples of any vomit for hospital analysis.*

Burns

Cool the burn

- Cool the burn immediately with cold *(preferably running)* water for 10 minutes or until the pain is relieved.
- If water is not available, any cold harmless liquid *(e.g. milk)* is better than no cooling at all. Do this first then move quickly to a water supply to continue cooling the burn.
- Take care not to cool large areas of burns so much that you induce hypothermia.

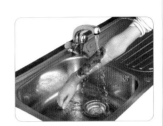

Remove jewellery and loose clothing

- Remove any constricting items, such as rings and watches if possible, because the area may start to swell.
- Carefully remove loose clothing, taking care that it's not stuck to the burn. *(If the burns are caused by chemicals be careful not to contaminate yourself or other areas of the casualty's body).*
- Leave clothing in place if you're not sure that it's loose.

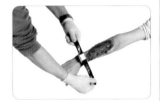

Dress the burn

- Dress the burn with a sterile dressing that won't stick. Cling film is one of the best dressings for a burn – discard the first two turns from the roll and apply it lengthways *(don't wrap it tightly around a limb)*. Secure with a bandage.
- Alternative dressings could be a new, unused plastic bag, low adherent dressings or specialised burns dressings *(do not rely on burns dressings to cool a burn – use cold water)*.
- See note *(below right)* on when to seek medical advice.
- If the burn appears severe, or the casualty has breathed in smoke or fumes, **call 999/112 for emergency help**.

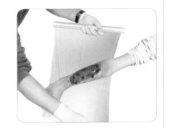

NEVER:

- Burst blisters.
- Touch the burn.
- Apply lotions, ointments or fats.
- Apply adhesive tape or dressings.
- Remove clothing that has stuck to the burn.

Seek medical advice if:

- *The burn is larger than 1-inch square.*
- *The casualty is a child.*
- *The burn goes all the way around a limb.*
- *Any part of the burn appears to be full thickness.*
- *The burn involves hands, feet, genitals or the face.*
- *You are not sure.*

Broken bones

Some signs and symptoms of a broken bone are:

Pain	At the site of the injury. Other injuries, nerve damage, or pain killers may mask the pain, so beware.
Loss of Power	For example not being able to lift anything with a fractured arm.
Unnatural movement	This type of fracture is classed as 'unstable' and care should be taken to prevent the bones from moving.
Swelling or bruising	Around the site of the injury.
Deformity	If a leg is bent in the wrong place, it's broken!
Irregularity	Lumps or depressions along the surface of the skin, where the broken ends of the bone overlap.
Crepitus	This is the feeling or sound of bone grating on bone if the broken ends rub on each other when the injury is moved about.
Tenderness	At the site of the injury.

Treatment of a broken bone

- Keep the injury still and the casualty warm.
- **Call 999/112 for emergency help if:**
  - There is a suspected injury to the spine, head or neck.
  - The casualty has difficulty breathing.
  - There is deformity, irregularity or unnatural movement.
  - The bone has come through the skin (or it looks as if it might do!).
  - The casualty seems to be in a lot of pain.
  - You can't easily get the casualty to hospital whilst keeping the injury still.
- Don't try bandaging the injury if you have called for an ambulance – just keep it still (gently cover open wounds with a sterile dressing).
- If you can easily get the casualty to hospital without moving the injury (and don't need an ambulance), gently support the injury and immobilise it if you can.

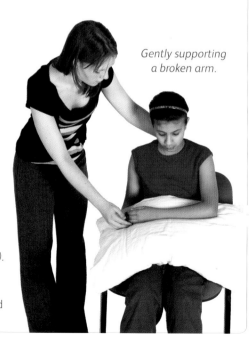

Gently supporting a broken arm.

Spinal injury

You should suspect spinal injury if the casualty has:

- Sustained a blow to the head, neck or back *(especially resulting in unconsciousness)*.
- Fallen from a height *(e.g. a fall from a horse)*.
- Dived into shallow water.
- Been in an accident involving speed *(e.g. knocked down or a car accident)*.
- Been involved in a 'cave in' accident *(e.g. crushing, or collapsed rugby scrum)*.
- Multiple injuries.
- Pain or tenderness in the neck or back after an accident *(beware – pain killers or other severe injuries may mask the pain)*.

If you are in any doubt, treat the casualty as if they have a spinal injury.

Treatment of spinal injury

If the casualty is conscious:

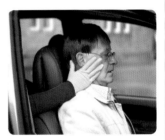

- Reassure the casualty. Tell them not to move.
- Keep the casualty in the position you find them. Do not allow them to move, unless they are in severe danger.
- Hold their head still with your hands. Keep the head and neck in line with the upper body *(see picture)*.
- **Call 999/112 for emergency help**. Keep the casualty still and warm until it arrives.

Keeping the head still in a car.

If the casualty is unconscious:

- If the casualty is breathing normally this means the airway must be clear, so there is no need to tip the head back *(you may have to gently tip it back and resuscitate if they are not!)*.
- **Call 999/112 for emergency help.**
- Hold the head still with your hands. Keep the head and neck in line with the upper body *(see picture)*.
- If you have to **leave** the casualty, if they begin to **vomit**, or if you are concerned about their **airway** in any way, you should put them into the **recovery position. Keep the head and neck in line with the spine whilst you turn the casualty.** Get help doing this if you can.
- Keep the casualty warm and still. Constantly monitor breathing until help arrives. Only move the casualty if they are in severe danger.

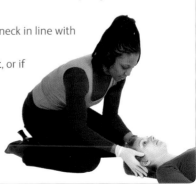

Heart attack

Some of the common signs and symptoms of a heart attack are listed below, but only a few might be present:

- A 'vice-like' pain in the centre of the chest, often described as 'tight' or 'a pressure' on the chest (can be mistaken for indigestion).
- The pain can sometimes spread into either arm (more commonly the left), the neck, jaw, back or shoulders.
- Pale, cold and clammy skin, sometimes with grey or blueness at the lips.
- The pulse can vary depending on the attack, sometimes missing beats (but it could just be normal!).
- Nausea or vomiting (feeling or being sick).
- Severe sweating.
- Shortness of breath.
- Dizziness or weakness.

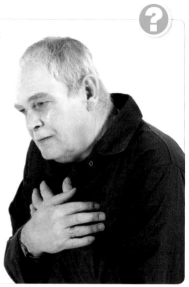

Treatment of heart attack

- Sit the casualty down and make them comfortable. A half sitting position is often the best (see picture). Don't allow them to walk around.
- **Call 999/112 for emergency help.**
- If the casualty suffers from angina, help them to take their angina medication (usually a spray or tablet for under the tongue).
- Reassure the casualty. Remove any causes of stress or anxiety if possible.
- If the casualty is not allergic to aspirin and older than 16, allowing them to **chew** an aspirin tablet **slowly** may help to limit the extent of damage to the heart.

NOTE: A first aider is not allowed to 'prescribe' drugs to a casualty. A fully conscious adult casualty is, however, more than capable of deciding whether or not they want to take medication that may help them.

- Monitor pulse and breathing.

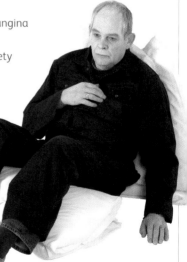

Stroke

There are two types of stroke. The most common is caused by a blood clot, blocking a blood vessel supplying part of the brain. The other is caused if a blood vessel in the brain ruptures, resulting in an area of the brain being 'squashed' by the pressure of the blood.

In either type of stroke, the signs and symptoms are very similar and an area of brain will die. A stroke can happen to a person of any age.

A stroke is a medical emergency. An urgent scan in hospital is required to find out the cause of the stroke, so that the correct treatment can be given quickly. The speed of treatment can have a dramatic impact on the casualty's recovery, but unfortunately it is often delayed because helpers call the doctor instead of calling 999.

Possible signs and symptoms

If you suspect stroke you should carry out the '**FAST**' test:

F Facial Weakness – can the person smile? Has their mouth or eye drooped?

A Arm Weakness – can the person raise both arms?

S Speech Problems – can the person speak clearly and understand what you say?

T Time to call 999/112 – if they fail any test, because stroke is a medical emergency.

Other signs and symptoms to look for include:

- Sudden numbness of the face or one side of the body.
- Loss of balance.
- Lack of coordination.
- Sudden severe headache.
- Sudden onset of confusion.
- Sight problems in one or both eyes.
- Unequal pupil size *(see pictures)*.

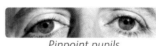
Pinpoint pupils

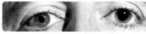
Unequal pupils

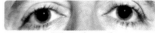
Dilated pupils

Treatment of stroke

- Maintain **Airway** and **Breathing** *(pages 4–6)*.
- **Call 999/112 for emergency help.**
- Place an unconscious casualty in the recovery position *(page 10)*.
- Lay the conscious casualty down, with head and shoulders raised.
- Reassure the casualty – do not assume that they don't understand.
- Monitor and record breathing, pulse and levels of response.

Diabetes

Diabetes is a condition suffered by a person who does not produce enough of a hormone called insulin.

Insulin works in your blood stream to 'burn off' the sugars that you eat. Some diabetics have such a lack of insulin, that they need to have insulin injections to keep their sugar levels down. This type of diabetic is called an 'insulin dependent' diabetic.

An insulin dependent diabetic has to make sure that they eat the right amount of sugar to match the insulin that they have injected. If they don't eat enough sugar *(by missing a meal for example)* the insulin injection will carry on burning off the small amount of sugar left in their blood stream, so their sugar levels may drop dangerously low.

Low blood sugar is dangerous because brain cells, unlike other cells in the body, can only use glucose *(sugar)* as their energy supply, so the brain is literally starved.

There are three common causes for a diabetic patients sugar levels to become low:

- *Missing a meal.*
- *Over exercising.*
- *Insulin overdose.*

Signs and symptoms of low blood sugar

- The condition usually starts and gets worse suddenly.
- Bizarre, uncharacteristic, uncooperative, possibly violent behaviour. Could be mistaken for 'drunkenness'.
- Confusion, memory loss.
- The casualty will deteriorate into unconsciousness if untreated.

- Pale, cold, sweaty skin.
- Shallow, rapid breathing and fast pulse.
- A diabetic casualty may carry an insulin pen, glucose tablets, a warning card, or wear a medic-alert bracelet or necklace.

DO NOT attempt to give the casualty anything to eat or drink if they become unconscious.

Treatment of low blood sugar

- Give the casualty a sugary drink *(isotonic sports drinks are best)*, sugar lumps, glucose tablets, or other sweet foods.
- If they respond to treatment quickly, give them more food or drink. Stay with them until they know what month it is.
- If they do not respond to treatment within 10 minutes, or they are unmanageable, **call 999/112 for emergency help.**
- Consider if there is another cause for the casualty's symptoms.
- **If the casualty becomes unconscious,** maintain **Airway** and **Breathing** *(pages 4–6)*, place them in the recovery position *(page 10)* and **call 999/112 for emergency help.**

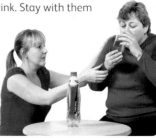

Seizures *(also known as fits or convulsions)*

There are many things that can cause a seizure, such as epilepsy, a lack of oxygen to the brain, a stroke *(a blood clot in the brain)*, a head injury, or even the body's temperature becoming too high *(this is common with babies and young children)*.

A major seizure often goes through a pattern:

'Tonic' Phase — Every muscle in the body becomes rigid. The casualty may let out a cry and will fall to the floor. The back may arch and the lips may go blue. This phase typically lasts less than 30 seconds.

'Clonic' Phase — The limbs of the body make sudden, violent jerking movements, the eyes may roll, the teeth may clench, saliva may drool from the mouth *(sometimes blood-stained as a result of biting the tongue)* and breathing could be loud like 'snoring'. The casualty may lose control of the bladder or bowel. This phase typically lasts less than 2 minutes.

Recovery Phase — The seizure stops and the casualty may go into a deep sleep, or become confused or agitated. They should come around within a few minutes.

Treatment of seizure

During the seizure

- Move dangerous objects away from the casualty.
- Gently protect the head with a folded coat or your hands.
- Time the seizure – make a note of the exact time and duration.
- Loosen any tight clothing around the neck to help breathing.
- **Call 999/112 for emergency help if:** the seizure lasts longer than 3 minutes, they have a second seizure, they have injured themselves, this is the casualty's first ever seizure, or the seizure lasts 2 minutes longer than is 'normal' for the casualty.

After the seizure

- Check **Airway** and **Breathing** *(pages 4–6)*.
- Place the casualty in the recovery position *(page 10)*.
- Move bystanders away before they wake, to protect modesty.
- **Call 999/112 for emergency help** if you can't wake them up within 10 minutes.
- Constantly monitor **Airway** and **Breathing**.

NEVER place anything in the mouth.

NEVER try to restrain the casualty.

NEVER move the casualty unnecessarily.

Asthma

Asthma is a condition caused by an allergic reaction in the lungs, often to substances such as dust, traffic fumes or animal hair.

Muscles surrounding the tiny wind pipes in the lungs go into spasm and constrict, making it very difficult for the casualty to breathe.

Most asthma patients carry medication with them, usually in the form of an inhaler. Ask the casualty, but usually the blue inhaler is for 'emergency' use, opening the wind pipes to relieve the condition.

An asthma attack is a traumatic experience for the casualty, especially a child, so reassurance and a calm approach from the first aider is essential.

Possible signs and symptoms

- Difficulty breathing.
- Wheezy breath sounds originating from the lungs.
- Difficulty speaking (*will need to take a breath in the middle of a sentence*).
- Pale, clammy skin.
- Grey or blue lips and skin (*if the attack is very severe*).
- Use of muscles in the neck and upper chest when breathing.
- Exhaustion in a severe attack.
- May become unconscious and stop breathing in a prolonged attack.

Treatment of asthma attack

- Help the casualty to sit upright, leaning on a table or chair if necessary.
- Help the casualty to use their reliever inhaler. This can be repeated every few minutes if the attack does not ease.
- Try to take the casualty's mind off the attack – be calm, reassuring and make light conversation.
- If the attack is prolonged, severe, appears to be getting worse, or the casualty is becoming exhausted; **call 999/112 for emergency help.**
- Cold winter air can make an attack worse so don't take the casualty outside for fresh air!
- Keep the casualty upright – even if they become too weak to sit up on their own. Only lay an asthma attack casualty down if they become deeply unconscious.

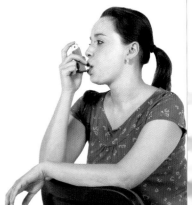

Allergic reaction *(anaphylaxis)*

Anaphylaxis is an extremely dangerous allergic reaction. The condition is caused by a massive over-reaction of the body's immune system.

Severe anaphylactic reactions are very rare, but if the airway or breathing are affected, death can occur in minutes.

Common allergies are to drugs *(such as penicillin)*, peanuts, egg or milk products, insect stings or seafoods.

The main chemical that the immune cells release if they detect a 'foreign protein' is called **'histamine'**. It is the massive quantities of histamine being released in the body during an anaphylactic reaction that cause the signs and symptoms of the condition:

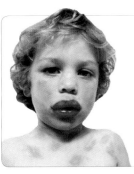

Signs and symptoms

- Swelling of the face, tongue, lips, neck and eyes.
- Difficulty breathing *(the casualty may have the equivalent of an asthma attack as well as a swollen airway).*
- Fast, weak pulse.
- Red, blotchy rash on the skin.
- Anxiety.

Picture: many thanks to the Anaphylaxis Campaign. www.anaphylaxis.org.uk © MedicalMediaKits.com

Treatment of anaphylaxis

- **Call 999/112 for emergency help.**
- Lay the casualty in a comfortable position:
  - If the casualty has Airway or Breathing problems they may prefer to sit up as this will make breathing easier.
  - **If the casualty feels faint however – do not sit them up.**
    Lay them down immediately. Raise the legs if they still feel faint.
- The casualty may have been issued an auto-injector of adrenaline. This can save their life if it's given promptly. The casualty should be able to inject this on their own but, if necessary, assist them to use it.
- If the casualty becomes unconscious – check **Airway** and **Breathing** *(pages 4–6)* and resuscitate as necessary.
- The dose of adrenaline can be repeated at 5 minute intervals if there is no improvement or symptoms return.

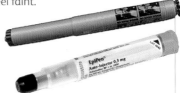

'EpiPen' and 'Anapen' are types of adrenaline auto-injectors.

Employer's responsibilities

Under Health and Safety law, an employer has a responsibility to ensure that first aid provision in the workplace is sufficient. This includes:

- Carrying out an assessment to decide how many first aiders are needed and where they should be located, following guidance from the Heath and Safety Executive.
- Providing training and re-qualifying training for their first aiders.
- Providing sufficient first aid kits and equipment for the workplace.
- Ensuring that all staff are aware of how and where to get first aid treatment.

Further information on first aid at work regulations can be found on the Health and Safety Executive website: **www.hse.gov.uk**

First aid kits

First aid kits should be easily accessible and clearly identified by a white cross on a green background. The container should protect the contents from dust and damp. A first aid kit should be available at every work site. Larger sites may need more than one first aid kit. The following list of contents is given as guidance:

1   leaflet giving general guidance on first aid.

20   individually wrapped plasters of assorted size. Blue detectable plasters should be provided for food handlers.

2   sterile eye pads.

4   triangular bandages, individually wrapped and preferably sterile.

6   safety pins.

6   medium wound dressings *(approx. 12cm x 12cm)*, individually wrapped and sterile.

2   large wound dressings *(approx. 18cm x 18cm)*.

1   pair of disposable gloves.

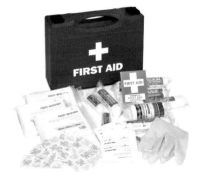

This list is not mandatory, so equivalent items may be used. Other items such as scissors, adhesive tape or disposable aprons should be provided if necessary. They may be stored in the first aid kit if they will fit, or kept close by for use.

Eye wash

If mains tap water is not readily available for eye irrigation, at least 1 litre of sterile water or 'saline' should be provided in sealed disposable container(s).

Notes

Notes

Notes

Notes